Lung Health

Tips and Strategies to Breathe Better and Live Longer

Watchman Amos

Table of contents

Introduction

Welcome to the book "Lungs Care: Making Your Lungs Always Active and Alive". In this book, you will learn how to take care of your lungs, one of the most vital organs in your body. Your lungs are responsible for breathing, which is the process of taking in oxygen and removing carbon dioxide. Oxygen is essential for every cell in your body to function properly, and carbon dioxide is a waste product that needs to be eliminated. Breathing also helps regulate your blood pressure, heart rate, and temperature. Without healthy lungs, you cannot live a healthy life.

However, many people neglect their lung health and take it for granted. According to the World Health Organization, lung diseases are among the leading causes of death and disability worldwide. Some of the common lung diseases include asthma, chronic obstructive pulmonary disease (COPD), lung cancer, tuberculosis, pneumonia, and COVID-19. These diseases can affect your quality of life, limit your activities, and shorten your lifespan. They can also impose a huge burden on the health care system and the economy.

The good news is that many lung diseases are preventable or manageable. You can do a lot to keep your lungs healthy and prevent or reduce the risk of lung problems. The main goal of this book is to provide you with practical tips and strategies to achieve this goal. You will learn how to:

- Not smoke or vape, and quit if you do
- Avoid exposure to air pollutants, both indoors and outdoors
- Get regular check-ups and screenings for lung diseases
- Be physically active and exercise your lungs

- Maintain a very healthy diet and stay
  always hydrated
- Stay updated with vaccinations for
  respiratory infections

Each chapter of this book will cover one of
these topics in detail, and explain why and
how they are important for your lung health.
You will also find examples, stories, and
resources to help you apply the tips and
strategies in your daily life. By following the
advice in this book, you will be able to make
your lungs always active and alive, and
enjoy the benefits of having healthy lungs
for your overall well-being.

Chapter 1

Don't Smoke or Vape

Smoking and vaping are both harmful habits that can damage your lungs and your body in many ways. Here are some of the harmful effects of smoking and vaping:

Smoking and vaping can cause inflammation in your lungs, which means your lungs become swollen and irritated. This can make it harder for you to breathe and increase your risk of infections and asthma .
Smoking and vaping can narrow your air passages, which means your lungs have less space to take in oxygen and get rid of carbon dioxide. This can make you feel short of breath and reduce your lung capacity .
Smoking and vaping can destroy your lung tissue, which means your lungs lose their elasticity and ability to function properly. This can lead to chronic obstructive

pulmonary disease (COPD), which is a
group of lung diseases that cause breathing
difficulties, coughing, wheezing, and mucus
production .
Smoking and vaping can increase your risk
of lung cancer, which is a type of cancer that
starts in the cells of your lungs and can
spread to other parts of your body. Lung
cancer is one of the most common and
deadly cancers in the world, and smoking is
the main cause of it .

As you can see, smoking and vaping are
very bad for your health and can cause
serious and irreversible damage to your
lungs and your body. But the good news is
that you can quit smoking or vaping and
improve your health and your life. Here are
some tips on how to quit smoking or vaping:

- Set a "quit" date and stick to it.
  Choose a day that is meaningful to
  you, such as your birthday,
  anniversary, or New Year's Day. Mark

it on your calendar and tell your good friends and family about it. This will help you prepare mentally and emotionally for your quit journey.

- Find support from others who are quitting or have quit smoking or vaping. You can join a support group, call a quitline, use an app, or talk to a counsellor. You can also ask your friends and family to encourage you and help you stay on track. Having support from others can make a big difference in your success.

- Use nicotine replacement products, such as patches, gums, lozenges, inhalers, or sprays. These products can help you cope with the physical withdrawal symptoms of nicotine, such as cravings, irritability, anxiety, and mood swings. They can also reduce the temptation to smoke or vape when you are in a stressful or challenging situation.

- Avoid triggers that make you want to smoke or vape, such as alcohol, coffee, certain foods, or places where people smoke or vape. Try to change your habits and routines, such as drinking water instead of alcohol, chewing gum instead of smoking, or taking a walk instead of vaping. You can also remove any reminders of smoking or vaping from your home, car, or workplace, such as ashtrays, lighters, cigarettes, or e-cigarettes.

- Cope with cravings and withdrawal symptoms by using healthy and positive strategies, such as deep breathing, meditation, exercise, hobbies, or music. You can also distract yourself by calling a friend, reading a book, playing a game, or doing something else that you enjoy.

Remember that cravings and withdrawal symptoms are temporary and will fade over time. You can also reward yourself for your progress and achievements, such as buying yourself a gift, treating yourself to a movie, or celebrating with your loved ones.

Quitting smoking or vaping can be hard, but it is worth it. Here are some of the benefits of quitting smoking or vaping:

You will improve your lung function and reduce your risk of lung diseases, such as COPD and lung cancer. Your lungs will start to heal and repair themselves within hours of quitting, and you will notice that you can breathe easier and have more energy. You will save money that you would otherwise spend on cigarettes or e-cigarettes. Depending on how much you smoke or vape, you could save hundreds or thousands of dollars per year. You can use

that money for other things that are
important to you, such as paying off debts,
saving for a vacation, or donating to a
charity.
You will enhance your quality of life and
well-being. You will smell better, have
fresher breath, and have cleaner teeth and
gums. You will also have a better sense of
taste and smell, and enjoy your food more.
You will feel more confident, proud, and
happy about yourself and your
achievements.

Many people have quit smoking or vaping
and have changed their lives for the better.
Here are some success stories of people
who quit smoking or vaping and how it
improved their health and their life:

- John, 45, quit smoking after 25 years
  of smoking a pack a day. He was
  diagnosed with COPD and had trouble
  breathing and walking. He decided to
  quit smoking for his health and his

family. He used nicotine patches and joined a support group. He also started exercising and eating healthier. He has been smoke-free for two years and has improved his lung function and his fitness. He can now run a 5K and play with his kids without getting tired. He says quitting smoking was the best decision he ever made.

- Lisa, 32, quit vaping after 10 years of vaping every day. She was addicted to nicotine and had anxiety and insomnia. She decided to quit vaping for her mental health and her career. She used nicotine lozenges and talked to a counsellor. She also learned to meditate and relax. She has been vape-free for six months and has reduced her anxiety and improved her sleep. She can now focus better and perform better at work. She says quitting vaping was a liberating experience.

- Sam, 28, quit smoking and vaping after 12 years of using both. He was spending a lot of money and time on cigarettes and e-cigarettes. He decided to quit smoking and vaping for his financial and personal goals. He used nicotine sprays and an app. He also set a budget and a plan. He has been smoke-free and vape-free for one year and has saved over $3000. He can now afford to travel and pursue his hobbies. He says quitting smoking and vaping was a rewarding journey.

These are just some examples of how quitting smoking or vaping can change your life for the better. You can also quit smoking or vaping and enjoy the benefits of a healthier and happier life. You have the power and the potential to quit smoking or vaping. All you need is the motivation and the determination to do it. You are not alone

in this. You have the support and the
resources to help you. You can do it. You
can quit smoking or vaping. You can start
today. You can make it happen. You can be
a quitter. A winner. A success story..

Chapter 2

Avoid Exposure to Air Pollutants

Air pollution is the presence of harmful substances in the air that can damage the lungs and cause respiratory problems. Some of the common sources and types of air pollutants are:

Secondhand smoke This is the smoke that comes from burning tobacco products, such as cigarettes, cigars, or pipes, or the smoke that is exhaled by smokers. Secondhand smoke contains over 7,000 chemicals, many of which are carcinogenic (cancer-causing) or toxic. Secondhand smoke can irritate the lungs, worsen asthma, and increase the risk of lung cancer and other diseases.

Chemicals These are substances that are used or produced in various industries, such as manufacturing, agriculture, mining, or cleaning. Some examples of chemicals that can pollute the air are asbestos, benzene,

formaldehyde, lead, mercury, and
pesticides. Exposure to these chemicals can
cause inflammation, irritation, or scarring of
the lungs, as well as chronic diseases such
as bronchitis, emphysema, or cancer.

Mould This is a type of fungus that grows in
damp or humid places, such as bathrooms,
basements, or kitchens. Mould releases
spores and toxins into the air that can
trigger allergic reactions, asthma attacks, or
infections in the lungs. Some types of
mould, such as black mould, can also
produce mycotoxins, which are very harmful
to the lungs and other organs.

Radon This is a radioactive gas that is
naturally found in the soil and rocks. It can
seep into buildings through cracks or gaps
in the foundation, walls, or pipes. Radon is
odourless, colourless, and tasteless, so it is
hard to detect without a special test. Radon
is the second leading cause of lung cancer

after smoking, as it damages the DNA of the lung cells.

Dust This is a mixture of tiny particles that are suspended in the air, such as soil, sand, pollen, animal dander, or dust mites. Dust can irritate the lungs, cause coughing, sneezing, or wheezing, and trigger allergies or asthma. Some types of dust, such as silica or coal dust, can also cause serious lung diseases, such as silicosis or black lung.

Pollen This is a fine powder that is produced by plants for reproduction. Pollen can be carried by the wind or insects and enter the air. Pollen can cause hay fever, which is an allergic reaction that affects the nose, eyes, and throat. Pollen can also aggravate asthma or other respiratory conditions.

Outdoor air pollution This is the contamination of the air by various sources, such as vehicles, factories, power plants, fires, or volcanoes. Outdoor air pollution can include gases, such as carbon monoxide, nitrogen oxides, sulphur dioxide, or ozone, or particles, such as smoke, soot, or ash. Outdoor air pollution can reduce the oxygen level in the blood, inflame the airways, impair the lung function, and increase the risk of respiratory infections, asthma, chronic obstructive pulmonary disease (COPD), or lung cancer.

To protect the lungs from air pollution, it is important to improve the indoor air quality and avoid exposure to outdoor air pollution as much as possible. Here are some tips on how to do that:

Ventilate the rooms Opening the windows or doors can help to circulate the air and remove the pollutants. However, this should be done when the outdoor air quality is good, and not during peak traffic hours or when there is smoke or smog outside.

Use air filters Installing air filters or purifiers can help to capture the particles and allergens in the air and improve the indoor air quality. However, air filters should be cleaned or replaced regularly, as they can become clogged or contaminated over time.

Cleaning regularly Vacuuming, dusting, or mopping can help to reduce the dust and dirt in the house. However, cleaning products should be chosen carefully, as some of them can contain harsh chemicals or fragrances that can pollute the air. It is better to use natural or mild cleaners, such as vinegar, baking soda, or lemon juice.

Avoid scented products Candles, air fresheners, or perfumes can emit volatile organic compounds (VOCs), which are chemicals that can irritate the lungs or cause headaches, nausea, or dizziness. It is better to use unscented or natural products, such as essential oils, herbs, or flowers, to create a pleasant smell in the house.

Test for radon As radon is invisible and odourless, the only way to know if it is present in the house is to test for it. Radon test kits are available at hardware stores or online, and they are easy to use. If the radon level is high, it is advisable to contact a professional to fix the problem, such as sealing the cracks or installing a ventilation system.

Check the air quality index The air quality index (AQI) is a measure of how polluted the air is, based on the levels of various pollutants, such as ozone, particulate matter, or nitrogen dioxide. The AQI ranges from 1 to 500, with higher values indicating worse air quality. The AQI can be checked online or through mobile apps, and it can help to plan the outdoor activities accordingly.

Avoid exercising near high traffic areas
Vehicles are a major source of outdoor air pollution, as they emit exhaust fumes that contain harmful gases and particles. Exercising near high traffic areas can increase the intake of these pollutants and affect lung health. It is better to exercise in parks, trails, or other green spaces, away from the roads and traffic.

Wearing a mask can help to filter out some of the pollutants in the air and reduce the exposure to them. However, not all masks are equally effective, and some of them can be uncomfortable or restrictive. The best type of mask for protecting the lungs from air pollution is the N95 respirator, which can block 95% of the particles that are 0.3 microns or larger. However, these masks should be fitted properly and worn correctly, and they should be replaced when they become dirty or damaged.

Limit outdoor activities on bad air days
When the air quality is poor, it is advisable to limit the time spent outdoors, especially for people who have respiratory conditions, such as asthma, COPD, or allergies. Staying indoors can help to avoid the exposure to the pollutants and prevent the worsening of the symptoms. However, indoor air quality should also be maintained, as mentioned above.

Climate change and natural disasters can also affect lung health, as they can increase the frequency and intensity of events that can cause or worsen air pollution, such as wildfires, heat waves, and storms. Here are some of the effects and how to prepare for them:

Wildfires Wildfires can produce large amounts of smoke, which is a mixture of gases and particles that can irritate the eyes, nose, throat, and lungs. Smoke can also reduce visibility and create hazardous

driving conditions. Wildfires can be caused
by natural factors, such as lightning, or
human factors, such as arson or negligence.
To prepare for wildfires, it is important to
follow these steps:

- Create a fire-safe zone around the
  house, by clearing the vegetation,
  debris, or flammable materials that
  can fuel the fire.
- Have an emergency plan and kit, with
  essential items, such as water, food,
  medication, flashlight, radio, and
  mask.
- Stay informed about the fire situation
  and the evacuation orders, by
  listening to the local authorities or
  media.
- If advised to evacuate, do so
  immediately and follow the designated
  routes and shelters.
- If trapped by the fire, stay inside the
  house, close the doors and windows,
  and cover the gaps with wet towels or
  blankets.

- If exposed to smoke, seek medical attention if experiencing symptoms, such as coughing, wheezing, chest pain, or difficulty breathing.

Heat waves Heat waves are periods of abnormally high temperatures that can last for several days or weeks. Heat waves can increase the formation of ozone, which is a gas that can damage the lung tissue and cause inflammation, coughing, or shortness of breath. Heat waves can also cause dehydration, heat exhaustion, or heat stroke, which are conditions that can affect the body's ability to regulate the temperature and the blood pressure. To prepare for heat waves, it is important to follow these steps:

Stay hydrated, by drinking plenty of water and avoiding alcohol, caffeine, or sugary drinks that can dehydrate the body.

Stay cool, by wearing light and loose clothing, using fans or air conditioners, and avoiding direct sunlight or strenuous activities.

Stay informed, by checking the temperature and the heat index, which is a measure of how hot it feels, based on the temperature and the humidity.

Seek medical attention, if experiencing symptoms, such as dizziness, nausea, headache, or confusion, which can indicate heat-related illnesses.

Storms Storms are the result of atmospheric instability, when warm and moist air rises and meets cold and dry air. The rising air cools and condenses, forming clouds and precipitation. The difference in air pressure and temperature creates strong winds, which can rotate and produce thunderstorms or tornadoes. Storms can bring beneficial rain or destructive hail, depending on the size and shape of the ice crystals that form in the clouds.

Chapter 3

Get Regular Check-ups

Getting regular check-ups is important to prevent or detect lung diseases early, when they are easier to treat. Lung diseases are conditions that affect the function or structure of the lungs, such as asthma, COPD, pneumonia, tuberculosis, lung cancer, or pulmonary fibrosis. Lung diseases can cause serious complications, such as respiratory failure, heart problems, or death, if left untreated or unmanaged.

Some of the common signs and symptoms of lung diseases are:

Shortness of breath This is the feeling of not being able to breathe enough or comfortably. Shortness of breath can occur during exercise, stress, or exposure to allergens or pollutants, or it can be persistent and interfere with daily activities. Shortness of breath can indicate a problem with the lungs, such as asthma, COPD, or pulmonary embolism, or a problem with the heart, such as heart failure or arrhythmia.

Coughing This is the reflex action of clearing the throat or lungs of mucus, irritants, or foreign substances. Coughing can be acute or chronic, productive or dry, and vary in frequency and intensity. Coughing can be caused by infections, allergies, asthma, COPD, GERD, or lung cancer, among other conditions.

Wheezing This is the high-pitched whistling sound that is made when breathing, especially when exhaling. Wheezing can indicate a narrowing or obstruction of the airways, such as in asthma, bronchitis, or anaphylaxis, or a foreign body in the lungs, such as a tumour or a piece of food.

Chest pain This is the pain or discomfort that is felt in the chest area, which can be sharp, dull, burning, or squeezing. Chest pain can have many causes, some of which are related to the lungs, such as pneumonia, pleurisy, or lung cancer, and some of which are related to the heart, such as angina, heart attack, or pericarditis.

Blood in the sputum This is the presence of blood or blood-streaked mucus that is coughed up from the lungs or throat. Blood in the sputum can be a sign of a serious lung condition, such as tuberculosis, bronchiectasis, or lung cancer, or a bleeding disorder, such as haemophilia or anticoagulant use.

If any of these signs or symptoms are severe, persistent, or unusual, it is advisable to see a doctor for a proper diagnosis and treatment. Some of the common tests and procedures that are used to diagnose and monitor lung diseases are:

Chest X-ray This is a type of imaging test that uses a small amount of radiation to produce a picture of the chest, including the lungs, heart, ribs, and diaphragm. A chest X-ray can show the size, shape, and position of the lungs, and detect any abnormalities, such as infections, fluid, tumours, or fractures.

Spirometry This is a type of lung function test that measures how much and how fast the air can be inhaled and exhaled. A spirometer is a device that is connected to a mouthpiece, which the patient has to blow into. A spirometry can show the amount of air that can be held in the lungs, the amount of air that can be exhaled in one second, and the ratio between the two. A spirometry can diagnose and monitor conditions that affect the airflow, such as asthma, COPD, or bronchitis.

Blood tests These are tests that analyse the blood sample that is taken from a vein or a finger. Blood tests can measure the levels of various substances in the blood, such as oxygen, carbon dioxide, haemoglobin, or antibodies. Blood tests can indicate the oxygen and carbon dioxide exchange in the lungs, the presence of infections or inflammation, or the exposure to certain toxins or allergens.

Bronchoscopy This is a type of procedure that allows the doctor to look inside the airways and lungs, using a thin, flexible tube called a bronchoscope, which has a light and a camera at the end. The bronchoscope is inserted through the nose or mouth, and passed down the throat and into the lungs. A bronchoscopy can help to diagnose and treat conditions that affect the airways and lungs, such as infections, tumours, bleeding, or foreign bodies. A bronchoscopy can also be used to take samples of tissue or fluid for further analysis, or to deliver medication or other treatments to the lungs. Some of the common treatments and medications that are used to manage lung diseases are:

Inhalers These are devices that deliver
medication directly to the lungs, through a
spray, powder, or mist. Inhalers can be used
to treat or prevent symptoms of lung
diseases, such as asthma, COPD, or
allergies. Inhalers can contain different
types of medication, such as
bronchodilators, which relax the muscles
around the airways and open them up, or
corticosteroids, which reduce the
inflammation and swelling in the airways
and lungs.You will need to use your inhaler
correctly and regularly, as prescribed by
your doctor.

Oxygen therapy This is a treatment that
provides extra oxygen to the lungs, through
a mask, a nasal cannula, or a tube. Oxygen
therapy can be used to treat or prevent low
oxygen levels in the blood, which can occur
due to lung diseases, such as COPD,
pulmonary fibrosis, or pneumonia, or other
conditions, such as heart failure, anaemia,
or sleep apnea. Oxygen therapy can

improve the breathing, the energy, and the quality of life of the patients. You will need to use oxygen therapy as prescribed by your doctor, and follow the safety precautions, such as avoiding smoking or fire.

Antibiotics These are medications that kill or stop the growth of bacteria, which can cause infections in the lungs, such as pneumonia, tuberculosis, or bronchitis. Antibiotics can be taken orally, intravenously, or inhaled, depending on the type and severity of the infection. Antibiotics can help to clear the infection, reduce the fever, and prevent the complications or the spread of the disease. You will need to take antibiotics as prescribed by your doctor, and complete the full course, even if you're feeling better.

Steroids These are medications that mimic the effects of hormones, such as cortisol, which are produced by the adrenal glands. Steroids can be taken orally, intravenously, or inhaled, depending on the type and severity of the condition. Steroids can help to reduce the inflammation, the swelling, and the immune response in the lungs, which can occur due to lung diseases, such as asthma, COPD, or sarcoidosis, or other conditions, such as autoimmune disorders, or allergic reactions. Steroids can help to improve the breathing, the lung function, and the symptoms of the patients.

Surgery This is a type of procedure that involves making an incision and removing or repairing a part of the body. Surgery can be used to treat or prevent lung diseases, such as lung cancer, pulmonary embolism, or pneumothorax, or other conditions, such as chest trauma, or congenital defects. Surgery can help to remove the diseased or damaged tissue, restore the normal function of the lungs, or improve the survival or the quality of life of the patients.
It can also be used to remove part or all of your lung, or to transplant a healthy lung

from a donor. Surgery can be open or minimally invasive, depending on the type and extent of the operation. You will need to undergo surgery as recommended by your doctor, and follow the preoperative and postoperative care, such as fasting, taking medication, or doing exercises.

Chapter 4

Be Physically Active

Physical activities are any movement that makes your muscles work and requires your body to burn calories. It can have many benefits for your lung health, such as:

- Strengthening the respiratory muscles: Physical activity can improve the endurance and efficiency of the muscles that help you breathe, such as the diaphragm, the intercostal muscles, and the abdominal muscles. This can help you breathe deeper and easier, and reduce the work of breathing.
- Improving the oxygen delivery: Physical activity can increase the blood flow and the oxygen delivery to your lungs and other organs. This can help your lungs exchange oxygen and carbon dioxide more effectively, and

improve your oxygen saturation and utilisation.
- Clearing the airways: Physical activity can help you cough up and clear the mucus and secretions that may accumulate in your airways, especially if you have a chronic lung disease, such as bronchitis or cystic fibrosis. This can help you prevent infections, reduce inflammation, and improve your lung function.
- Boosting the immune system: Physical activity can stimulate the production and activity of the white blood cells and the antibodies that fight against germs and diseases. This can help you prevent or recover from respiratory infections, such as the common cold, the flu, or pneumonia.

To start and maintain a regular exercise routine, you can follow these guidelines:
- Choose an activity that is enjoyable: Physical activity can be fun and

rewarding, if you choose something that you like and that suits your preferences, abilities, and goals. You can try different types of activities, such as aerobic, anaerobic, or flexibility exercises, and find out what works best for you. You can also vary your routine, to avoid boredom and monotony.

- Set realistic goals: Physical activity can be challenging and rewarding, if you set goals that are specific, measurable, achievable, relevant, and time-bound. You can start with small and easy goals, such as walking for 10 minutes a day, and gradually increase the intensity, duration, and frequency of your exercise, as you improve your fitness and confidence. You can also track your progress, by using a diary, a calendar, or an app, and celebrate your achievements, by

rewarding yourself or sharing with
others.

- Warm up and cool down: Physical
  activity can be safe and effective, if
  you prepare your body and mind
  before and after your exercise. You
  can warm up, by doing some light and
  gentle movements, such as stretching,
  jogging, or skipping, for 5 to 10
  minutes, to increase your blood
  circulation, heart rate, and muscle
  temperature. You can also cool down,
  by doing some slow and relaxing
  movements, such as walking,
  breathing, or meditating, for 5 to 10
  minutes, to lower your blood pressure,
  heart rate, and muscle tension.

- Listen to your body: Physical activity
  can be enjoyable and beneficial, if you
  listen to your body and respect your
  limits. You can use the **Borg scale**
  to monitor your perceived exertion,

which is how hard you feel your exercise is, on a scale from 0 to 10, where 0 is nothing at all, and 10 is very, very hard. You can aim for a moderate level of exertion, which is around 4 to 6, where you can talk but not sing. You can also pay attention to your symptoms, such as shortness of breath, chest pain, dizziness, or fatigue, and stop or rest if you feel any discomfort or difficulty.

Some examples of exercises that are good for the lungs are:

Walking: This is a type of aerobic exercise that involves moving your feet and legs at a steady pace. It can improve your cardiovascular and respiratory fitness, and strengthen your muscles and bones. It can also be easy and convenient, as you can do it anywhere and anytime, such as in a park, a mall, or a treadmill. To perform walking safely and effectively, you can:

- Wear comfortable and supportive shoes and clothes.
- Maintain a good posture, with your head up, your shoulders back, and your arms swinging.
- Breathe deeply and rhythmically, through your nose and mouth, and exhale longer than you inhale.
- Start slowly and gradually, and increase your speed and distance, as you feel comfortable.
- Drink plenty of water, before, during, and after your walk.

Jogging: This is a type of aerobic exercise that involves running at a slow or moderate speed. It can improve your cardiovascular and respiratory fitness, and burn more calories and fat than walking. It can also be fun and challenging, as you can vary your pace, terrain, and distance, such as in a track, a road, or a trail. To perform jogging safely and effectively, you can:

- Wear comfortable and supportive shoes and clothes, and use a stopwatch or a music player to time your jog.
- Warm up and cool down, by walking for 5 to 10 minutes, before and after your jog.
- Breathe deeply and rhythmically, through your nose and mouth, and exhale longer than you inhale.
- Start slowly and gradually, and increase your speed and distance, as you feel comfortable.
- Drink plenty of water, before, during, and after your jogging.

Cycling: This is a type of aerobic exercise that involves pedalling a bicycle or a stationary bike. It can improve your cardiovascular and respiratory fitness, and strengthen your lower body muscles and joints. It can also be enjoyable and adventurous, as you can explore different routes and sceneries, such as in a park, a road, or a mountain. To perform cycling safely and effectively, you can:

- Wear comfortable and protective gear, such as a helmet, gloves, and sunglasses, and use a bike that fits your size and style.
- Maintain a good posture, with your back straight, your elbows slightly bent, and your knees aligned with your feet.
- Breathe deeply and rhythmically, through your nose and mouth, and exhale longer than you inhale.
- Start slowly and gradually, and increase your speed and resistance, as you feel comfortable.
- Drink plenty of water, before, during, and after your cycling.

Swimming: This is a type of aerobic exercise that involves moving your arms and legs in water. It can improve your cardiovascular and respiratory fitness, and tone your whole body muscles. It can also be relaxing and refreshing, as you can enjoy the water and the buoyancy, such as in a pool, a lake, or an ocean. To perform swimming safely and effectively, you can:

- Wear comfortable and appropriate swimwear and accessories, such as a swimsuit, goggles, and a cap, and use a pool that is clean and supervised.
- Choose a stroke that suits your skill and preference, such as freestyle, breaststroke, backstroke, or butterfly, and learn the proper technique and form.
- Breathe deeply and rhythmically, through your mouth and nose, and exhale longer than you inhale, and coordinate your breathing with your strokes.

- Start slowly and gradually, and increase your speed and distance, as you feel comfortable.
- Drink plenty of water, before, during, and after your swim.

Yoga: This is a type of flexibility exercise that involves doing various poses and movements, while focusing on your breathing and awareness. It can improve your lung capacity and function, and reduce your stress and anxiety. It can also be calming and soothing, as you can connect with your body and mind, such as in a studio, a home, or a garden. To perform yoga safely and effectively, you can:

- Wear comfortable and loose clothes, and use a mat, a cushion, or a blanket, and a quiet and comfortable space.
- Choose a style that suits your level and goal, such as hatha, vinyasa,

bikram, or ashtanga, and learn the proper technique and alignment.
- Breathe deeply and rhythmically, through your nose and mouth, and exhale longer than you inhale, and coordinate your breathing with your movements.
- Start slowly and gradually, and increase your intensity and duration, as you feel comfortable.
- Drink plenty of water, before, during, and after your yoga.

To overcome the barriers and challenges to physical activity, you can follow these tips:
- Lack of time: Physical activity can be integrated into your daily routine, if you plan ahead and prioritise your exercise. You can schedule your exercise, by setting a specific time and place, and sticking to it. You can also break your exercise, by doing short and frequent sessions, such as 10 minutes, three times a day, instead

of one long session. You can also use your spare time, such as during breaks, lunch, or commute, to do some physical activity, such as walking, stretching, or climbing stairs.

- Lack of motivation: Physical activity can be motivating and rewarding, if you find your purpose and passion for exercise. You can remind yourself of the benefits of exercise, such as improving your health, mood, and appearance. You can also set realistic and achievable goals, such as walking for 30 minutes a day, and track your progress and celebrate your achievements, by using a diary, a calendar, or an app. You can also find a partner or a group, such as a friend, a family member, or a club, to exercise with, and support and encourage each other.

- Lack of access: Physical activity can be accessible and affordable, if you use the resources and opportunities that are available and convenient for you. You can use your own body weight, or household items, such as cans, bottles, or books, as resistance tools, to do strength exercises, such as squats, lunges, or push-ups. You can also use your own environment, such as stairs, benches, or walls, as exercise equipment, to do cardio exercises, such as running, jumping, or climbing. You can also use online tools to access free or low-cost videos, programs, and guides that can help you exercise at home or anywhere.

- Discomfort or difficulty in breathing: Physical activity can be comfortable and manageable, if you adjust your exercise according to your condition and symptoms. You can use the *Borg scale* to monitor your perceived exertion, which is how hard you feel your exercise is, on a scale from 0 to 10, where 0 is nothing at all, and 10 is very, very hard. You can aim for a moderate level of exertion, which is around 4 to 6, where you can talk but not sing. You can also pay attention to your symptoms, such as shortness of breath, chest pain, dizziness, or fatigue, and stop or rest if you feel any discomfort or difficulty. You can also use your inhaler or oxygen therapy, if prescribed by your doctor, to help you breathe easier during exercise.

Chapter 5

Maintain a Healthy Diet and Stay Hydrated

Nutrition and hydration are essential for your lung health, as they play important roles in:

☐ Providing the energy and nutrients for the metabolism: Your lungs need energy and nutrients to perform their functions, such as breathing, gas exchange, and mucus clearance. The energy and nutrients come from the food and drinks that you consume, and are delivered to your lungs by your blood. The food and drinks that you consume also affect your blood pH, which is the measure of how acidic or alkaline your blood is. Your blood pH affects your breathing rate, as your lungs try to maintain a balance between the carbon dioxide and the oxygen in your blood. A balanced diet can help you provide enough energy and nutrients for your lungs, and keep your blood pH within the normal range.

☐ Supporting the immune system: Your lungs are exposed to various germs and pollutants that can cause infections and inflammations in your airways and lungs. Your immune system is your body's defence mechanism that fights against these harmful invaders, and protects your lungs from damage. The food and drinks that you consume can influence your immune system, as they contain various substances, such as vitamins, minerals, antioxidants, and phytochemicals, that can enhance or impair your immune response. A healthy diet can help you boost your immune system, and prevent or recover from respiratory infections.

☐ Thinning the mucus in the airways: Your lungs produce mucus, which is a sticky and slippery substance that lines your airways and lungs. Mucus helps you trap and remove the germs and pollutants that enter your lungs, and moisten and protect your airways and lungs. However, too much or too thick mucus can clog your airways and lungs, and make it harder for you to breathe. The food and drinks that you consume can affect the amount and the consistency of your mucus, as they can increase or decrease your mucus production, and make your mucus thicker or thinner. A balanced diet can help you thin your mucus in your airways, and make it easier for you to cough it up and clear it out.

To follow a healthy diet, you can follow these general principles:

Eat a variety of foods: Eating a variety of foods can help you get all the nutrients that your body and your lungs need, such as carbohydrates, proteins, fats, vitamins, minerals, and water. Eating a variety of foods can also help you prevent nutritional deficiencies or excesses, and enjoy different flavours and textures. You can eat a variety of foods, by choosing foods from different food groups, such as grains, fruits, vegetables, dairy, meat, eggs, nuts, seeds, and legumes, and eating different colours, shapes, and sizes of foods.

Limit the intake of salt, sugar, and fat: Eating too much salt, sugar, and fat can harm your health and your lungs, as they can increase your blood pressure, blood sugar, blood cholesterol, and body weight. High blood pressure, blood sugar, blood cholesterol, and body weight can increase your risk of developing various chronic diseases, such as diabetes, heart disease, stroke, and some types of cancer, which can affect your lung function and oxygen delivery. High salt intake can also increase your mucus production, and make your mucus thicker and harder to clear. You can limit your intake of salt, sugar, and fat, by choosing foods that are low in salt, sugar, and fat, such as fresh, frozen, or canned foods without added salt, sugar, or fat, and avoiding foods that are high in salt, sugar, and fat, such as processed, fried, or baked foods, and sweets, snacks, or sauces.

Choose whole grains, fruits, vegetables, lean proteins, and healthy fats: Eating whole grains, fruits, vegetables, lean proteins, and healthy fats can benefit your health and your lungs, as they can provide you with various nutrients that can support your lung function and immune system, such as fibre, antioxidants, anti-inflammatory agents, and omega-3 fatty acids. Fibre can help you lower your blood pressure, blood sugar, blood cholesterol, and body weight, and improve your bowel movements and digestion. Antioxidants can help you protect your cells and tissues from oxidative stress and damage, and prevent or reduce inflammation and infection in your lungs. Anti-inflammatory agents can help you reduce inflammation and swelling in your airways and lungs, and improve your breathing and gas exchange. Omega-3 fatty acids can help you lower your blood pressure, blood cholesterol, and inflammation, and improve your blood flow and oxygen delivery. You can choose whole grains, fruits, vegetables, lean proteins, and healthy fats, by choosing foods that are rich in these nutrients, such as whole wheat bread, brown rice, oats, quinoa, apples, berries, oranges, bananas, broccoli, spinach, carrots, tomatoes, chicken, fish, eggs, tofu, beans, lentils, nuts, seeds, olive oil, and avocado.

Some examples of foods that are good for the lungs are:

Apples: Apples are fruits that are rich in fibre, antioxidants, and phytochemicals, such as quercetin, catechin, and phloridzin. Apples can help you lower your blood pressure, blood sugar, blood cholesterol, and body weight, and improve your bowel movements and digestion. Apples can also help you protect your cells and tissues from oxidative stress and damage, and prevent or reduce inflammation and infection in your lungs. Apples can also help you thin your mucus in your airways, and make it easier for you to cough it up and clear it out.

Berries: Berries are fruits that are rich in fibre, antioxidants, and phytochemicals, such as anthocyanins, flavonoids, and ellagic acid. Berries can help you lower your blood pressure, blood sugar, blood cholesterol, and body weight, and improve your bowel movements and digestion. Berries can also help you protect your cells and tissues from oxidative stress and damage, and prevent or reduce inflammation and infection in your lungs. Berries can also help you boost your immune system, and prevent or recover from respiratory infections.

Broccoli: Broccoli is a vegetable that is rich in fibre, antioxidants, and phytochemicals, such as sulforaphane, indole-3-carbinol, and glucosinolates. Broccoli can help you lower your blood pressure, blood sugar, blood cholesterol, and body weight, and improve your bowel movements and digestion. Broccoli can also help you protect your cells and tissues from oxidative stress and damage, and prevent or reduce inflammation and infection in your lungs. Broccoli can also help you activate your immune system, and fight against germs and diseases.

Garlic: Garlic is a spice that is rich in antioxidants and phytochemicals, such as allicin, diallyl sulphide, and ajoene. Garlic can help you lower your blood pressure, blood sugar, blood cholesterol, and body weight, and improve your blood flow and oxygen delivery. Garlic can also help you protect your cells and tissues from oxidative stress and damage, and prevent or reduce inflammation and infection in your lungs. Garlic can also help you kill or inhibit the growth of bacteria, viruses, fungi, and parasites that cause respiratory infections, such as pneumonia, tuberculosis, or bronchitis.

Ginger: Ginger is a spice that is rich in antioxidants and phytochemicals, such as gingerol, shogaol, and zingerone. Ginger can help you lower your blood pressure, blood sugar, blood cholesterol, and body weight, and improve your blood flow and oxygen delivery. Ginger can also help you protect your cells and tissues from oxidative stress and damage, and prevent or reduce inflammation and infection in your lungs. Ginger can also help you relax and dilate your airways, and improve your breathing and gas exchange.

Turmeric: Turmeric is a spice that is rich in antioxidants and phytochemicals, such as curcumin, , and bisdemethoxycurcumin. Turmeric can help you lower your blood pressure, blood sugar, blood cholesterol, and body weight, and improve your blood flow and oxygen delivery. Turmeric can also help you protect your cells and tissues from oxidative stress and damage, and prevent or reduce inflammation and infection in your lungs. Turmeric can also help you modulate your immune system, and balance your inflammatory and anti-inflammatory responses.

To stay hydrated, you can always follow these tips:

Drink water throughout the day: Drinking water throughout the day can help you maintain your fluid balance, and prevent dehydration, which can affect your lung function and oxygen delivery. Drinking water throughout the day can also help you thin your mucus in your airways, and make it easier for you to cough it up and clear it out. You can drink water throughout the day, by drinking at least 8 glasses of water a day, or more if you exercise, sweat, or have a fever. You can also drink water before, during, and after your meals, and whenever you feel thirsty or dry.

Avoid caffeine and alcohol: Avoiding caffeine and alcohol can help you stay hydrated, as they can dehydrate you, by increasing your urine output, and reducing your fluid intake. Caffeine and alcohol can also affect your blood pressure, heart rate, and blood vessels, which can affect your lung function and oxygen delivery. Caffeine and alcohol can also irritate your airways and lungs, increase your mucus production, and make your mucus thicker and harder to clear. You can avoid caffeine and alcohol, by limiting or avoiding drinks that contain caffeine, such as coffee, tea, energy drinks, or cola, and drinks that contain alcohol, such as beer, wine, or liquor.

Eat foods with high water content: Eating foods with high water content can help you stay hydrated, as they can provide you with water and nutrients, and make you feel full and satisfied. Foods with high water content can also help you thin your mucus in your airways, and make it easier for you to cough it up and clear it out. You can eat foods with high water content, by choosing foods that are rich in water, such as fruits, vegetables, soups, salads, yoghurt, and milk. You can also eat foods that are rich in electrolytes, such as sodium, potassium, calcium, and magnesium, which can help you balance your fluid and pH levels, such as bananas, oranges, tomatoes, potatoes, spinach, cheese, and nuts.

Chapter 6

Stay Up to Date with Vaccinations

Vaccinations are a type of preventive medicine that can protect you from getting or spreading infectious respiratory diseases, such as influenza, COVID-19, pneumococcal pneumonia, and RSV, that can damage your lungs. Vaccinations work by stimulating your immune system to produce antibodies, which are proteins that can recognize and fight against specific germs that cause diseases. Vaccinations can help you prevent or reduce the severity of respiratory infections, and lower your risk of developing complications, such as bronchitis, asthma, or COPD.

The types and schedules of vaccinations that are recommended for different age groups and risk factors are:

Influenza vaccine: This is a vaccine that can protect you from the seasonal flu, which is a common and contagious respiratory infection caused by various strains of influenza viruses. The flu can cause symptoms such as fever, cough, sore throat, runny nose, headache, muscle ache, and fatigue, and can lead to serious complications, such as pneumonia, ear infections, sinus infections, or sepsis. The influenza vaccine is updated every year, based on the predicted strains of influenza viruses that will circulate in the upcoming flu season. The influenza vaccine is recommended for everyone 6 months and older, every year, preferably before the end of October. The influenza vaccine is especially important for people who are at high risk of developing severe flu or complications, such as children, older adults, pregnant women, and people with chronic conditions, such as diabetes, heart disease, lung disease, or immune system disorders.

COVID-19 vaccine: This is a vaccine that can protect you from COVID-19, which is a novel and pandemic respiratory infection caused by a new strain of coronavirus, called SARS-CoV-2. COVID-19 can cause symptoms such as fever, cough, shortness of breath, loss of taste or smell, headache, fatigue, and diarrhoea, and can lead to serious complications, such as pneumonia, blood clots, organ failure, or death. The COVID-19 vaccine is developed and authorised by various manufacturers, such as Pfizer-BioNTech, Moderna, Johnson & Johnson, AstraZeneca, and Sinovac, based on different technologies, such as mRNA, viral vector, or inactivated virus. The COVID-19 vaccine is recommended for everyone 12 years and older, depending on the availability and eligibility in your country or region. The COVID-19 vaccine is especially important for people who are at high risk of developing severe COVID-19 or complications, such as older adults, people with chronic conditions, health care workers, or essential workers.

Pneumococcal vaccine: This is a vaccine that can protect you from pneumococcal pneumonia, which is a serious and potentially fatal respiratory infection caused by a type of bacteria, called Streptococcus pneumoniae. Pneumococcal pneumonia can cause symptoms such as fever, cough, chest pain, difficulty breathing, and blood in the sputum, and can lead to complications, such as meningitis, septicemia, or otitis media. There are two types of pneumococcal vaccines, such as pneumococcal conjugate vaccine (PCV13), which protects against 13 types of pneumococcal bacteria, and pneumococcal polysaccharide vaccine (PPSV23), which protects against 23 types of pneumococcal bacteria. The pneumococcal vaccine is recommended for children under 5 years old, adults 65 years and older, and people with certain medical conditions, such as diabetes, heart disease, lung disease, or immune system disorders. The pneumococcal vaccine is given in different doses and intervals, depending on your age and risk factors.

RSV vaccine: This is a vaccine that can protect you from respiratory syncytial virus (RSV), which is a common and contagious respiratory infection that affects mostly infants and young children. RSV can cause symptoms such as runny nose, cough, wheezing, fever, and difficulty breathing, and can lead to complications, such as bronchiolitis, pneumonia, or asthma. There is no licensed RSV vaccine for the general population, but there is a preventive medication, called palivizumab, which is a type of antibody that can prevent severe RSV infection in high-risk infants and children, such as premature babies, babies with heart or lung problems, or babies with immune system disorders. Palivizumab is given as an injection, once a month, during the RSV season, which is usually from November to April.

To get vaccinated, you can follow these tips:

Find a nearby clinic: You can find a nearby clinic that offers the vaccinations that you need, by using online tools, such as [Vaccine Finder] or [Vax Locator], or by contacting your local health department, your healthcare provider, or your pharmacy. You can also check the availability and the cost of the vaccinations, and the insurance coverage and the payment options, before you visit the clinic.

Make an appointment: You can make an appointment for your vaccination, by calling the clinic, or by using online tools, such as [Vax Scheduler] or [Vaccine Spotter]. You can also check the requirements and the instructions for your appointment, such as the documents that you need to bring, the forms that you need to fill out, and the precautions that you need to take, such as wearing a mask, maintaining social distance, and avoiding contact with sick people.

Prepare for the visit: You can prepare for your visit, by doing some things that can make your vaccination more comfortable and effective, such as eating a healthy meal, drinking plenty of water, wearing loose and comfortable clothes, and bringing a friend or a family member for support. You can also prepare for your visit, by doing some things that can prevent or reduce the risk of adverse reactions, such as informing your health care provider of your medical history, your allergies, your medications, and your previous vaccinations, and asking any questions or concerns that you may have about the vaccination.

Follow the aftercare instructions: You can follow the aftercare instructions, by doing some things that can help you recover and monitor your health after your vaccination, such as resting, applying a cold compress, taking a pain reliever, and drinking plenty of water. You can also follow the aftercare instructions, by doing some things that can help you prevent or treat any side effects, such as fever, pain, swelling, redness, or itching at the injection site, or headache, fatigue, muscle ache, or nausea, and reporting any severe or persistent symptoms, such as difficulty breathing, chest pain, or allergic reaction, to your health care provider or emergency services.

The safety and effectiveness of vaccinations are:

- Possible side effects: Vaccinations are generally safe and well-tolerated, but

they may cause some mild and
temporary side effects, such as fever,
pain, swelling, redness, or itching at
the injection site, or headache,
fatigue, muscle ache, or nausea.
These side effects are normal and
expected, as they indicate that your
immune system is responding to the
vaccination, and they usually go away
within a few days, without any serious
consequences. However, in rare
cases, vaccinations may cause some
serious and life-threatening side
effects, such as difficulty breathing,
chest pain, or allergic reaction, which
require immediate medical attention.
These side effects are very
uncommon and unpredictable, and
they may occur due to various factors,
such as the type of vaccine, the dose
of vaccine, the individual's health
condition, or the individual's genetic
makeup.

- Benefits outweigh the risks:
  Vaccinations are effective and
  beneficial, as they can prevent or
  reduce the severity of infectious
  respiratory diseases that can spread
  from person to person and damage
  the lungs. Vaccinations can help you
  protect yourself and others from
  getting or spreading these diseases,
  and lower your risk of developing
  complications, such as bronchitis,
  asthma, or COPD. Vaccinations can
  also help you save time, money, and
  resources that would otherwise be
  spent on treating these diseases, and
  improve your quality of life and
  productivity. The benefits of
  vaccinations outweigh the risks of
  vaccinations, as the chances of
  getting or spreading these diseases,
  or developing complications, are much
  higher and more serious than the
  chances of experiencing side effects,
  or developing adverse reactions.

- Importance of herd immunity: Herd immunity is a phenomenon that occurs when a large proportion of a population is immune to a disease, either by vaccination or by natural infection, and can prevent or slow down the transmission of the disease to others, especially those who are not immune or vulnerable, such as infants, older adults, pregnant women, or people with

Conclusion

In this book, you have learned about the tips and strategies to breathe better and live longer, by taking care of your lung health. You have learned about the structure and function of your lungs, the common lung diseases and conditions, the risk factors and triggers that can harm your lungs, and the lifestyle and behavioural changes that can improve your lung health. You have also learned about the role of nutrition and hydration, physical activity, vaccinations, check-ups and tests, and treatments and medications, in supporting your lung health and preventing or managing lung problems.

The main purpose of this book is to help you understand the importance of your lung health, and how it affects your overall well-being. By following the advice and recommendations in this book, you can improve your lung function and capacity, reduce your symptoms and complications, and enhance your quality of life and longevity. You can also protect yourself and others from getting or spreading infectious respiratory diseases that can damage your lungs, and reduce the occurrence and the impact of outbreaks, epidemics, or pandemics.

We hope that you have enjoyed reading this book, and that you have gained some valuable knowledge and skills that you can apply in your daily lives. Remember that your lungs are vital organs that need your attention and care, and that you can take charge of your lung health, by making positive and proactive choices. You can also seek help and support from your doctor, your health care team, your family, and your friends, whenever you need it.

The main goal of this book is to help you keep your lungs healthy and prevent or manage lung problems, by providing you with the tips and strategies that are based on the latest scientific research and clinical practice. By following the advice and recommendations in this book, you can improve your lung function and capacity, reduce your symptoms and complications, and enhance your quality of life and longevity.

We hope that you have found this book useful and informative, and that you are motivated and encouraged to apply the tips and strategies in your daily lives. Remember that your lungs are vital organs that affect your overall well-being, and that you can take charge of your lung health, by making positive and proactive choices. You can also seek help and support from your doctor, your health care team, your family, and your friends, whenever you need it.

If you want to learn more about lung health and lung diseases, you can check out the following resources and references, that can provide you with more information and support:

American Lung Association: This is a national organisation that works to save lives by improving lung health and preventing lung disease, through research, education, and advocacy. It offers various programs and services, such as lung helpline, lung force, freedom from smoking, better breathers club, and asthma basics, and provides various resources and information, such as lung health tools, lung health topics, lung health research, and lung health news.

British Lung Foundation: This is a UK charity that works to support people affected by lung disease, and to improve lung health, through research, policy, and campaigning. It offers various services and support, such as helpline, web community, online forum, support groups, and events, and provides various resources and information, such as lung health advice, lung health stories, lung health publications, and lung health campaigns.

European Lung Foundation: This is a European organisation that works to bring together people who care about lung health, and to raise awareness of lung disease, through research, education, and communication. It offers various activities and initiatives, such as European respiratory society, breathe magazine, healthy lungs for life, and patient priorities, and provides various resources and information, such as lung health factsheets, lung health videos, lung health podcasts, and lung health newsletters.

Global Initiative for Chronic Obstructive Lung Disease (**GOLD**): This is a global organisation that works to improve the prevention and management of COPD, through collaboration with health care professionals and public health officials. It offers various guidelines and reports, such as global strategy for the diagnosis, management, and prevention of COPD, global strategy for asthma management and prevention, and global strategy for the prevention and control of tuberculosis, and provides various resources and information, such as COPD assessment test, COPD pocket guide, COPD slides, and COPD webinars.

World Health Organization (WHO): This is a global organisation that works to promote health, keep the world safe, and serve the vulnerable, through directing and coordinating international health within the United Nations system. It offers various programs and projects, such as universal health coverage, health emergencies, health and climate change, and health and human rights, and provides various resources and information, such as health topics, data and statistics, publications and reports, and news and events.

Thank you for your time and attention, and for choosing this book as your guide to lung health. We appreciate your feedback and experiences, and we invite you to share them with us, by contacting us at [prof.dr.gabjek@gmail.com], or by leaving a review on [Amazon]. We wish you all the best, and we hope that you breathe better and live longer.

9 798870 135953